Circadian Diet

A Beginner's 3-Week Step-by-Step Guide for Weight Loss and Health with Recipes and a Meal Plan

copyright © 2020 Bruce Ackerberg

All rights reserved No part of this book may be reproduced, or stored in a retrieval system, or transmitted in any form or by any means, electronic, mechanical, photocopying, recording, or otherwise, without express written permission of the publisher.

Disclaimer

By reading this disclaimer, you are accepting the terms of the disclaimer in full. If you disagree with this disclaimer, please do not read the guide.

All of the content within this guide is provided for informational and educational purposes only, and should not be accepted as independent medical or other professional advice. The author is not a doctor, physician, nurse, mental health provider, or registered nutritionist/dietician. Therefore, using and reading this guide does not establish any form of a physician-patient relationship.

Always consult with a physician or another qualified health provider with any issues or questions you might have regarding any sort of medical condition. Do not ever disregard any qualified professional medical advice or delay seeking that advice because of anything you have read in this guide. The information in this guide is not intended to be any sort of medical advice and should not be used in lieu of any medical advice by a licensed and qualified medical professional.

The information in this guide has been compiled from a variety of known sources. However, the author cannot attest to or guarantee the accuracy of each source and thus should not be held liable for any errors or omissions.

You acknowledge that the publisher of this guide will not be held liable for any loss or damage of any kind incurred as a result of this guide or the reliance on any information provided within this guide. You acknowledge and agree that you assume all risk and responsibility for any action you undertake in response to the information in this guide.

Using this guide does not guarantee any particular result (e.g., weight loss or a cure). By reading this guide, you acknowledge that there are no guarantees to any specific outcome or results you can expect.

All product names, diet plans, or names used in this guide are for identification purposes only and are the property of their respective owners. The use of these names does not imply endorsement. All other trademarks cited herein are the property of their respective owners.

Where applicable, this guide is not intended to be a substitute for the original work of this diet plan and is, at most, a supplement to the original work for this diet plan and never a direct substitute. This guide is a personal expression of the facts of that diet plan.

Where applicable, persons shown in the cover images are stock photography models and the publisher has obtained the rights to use the images through license agreements with third-party stock image companies.

Table of Contents

Introduction	**8**
What Is Circadian Rhythm?	**11**
How Circadian Rhythm Affects Metabolism	12
The Circadian Rhythm Diet	**14**
Principles of The Circadian Diet	16
The Benefits of the Circadian Rhythm Diet	18
Disadvantages of The Circadian Diet	20
How to Follow a Circadian Diet	**22**
Week 1: Assess your Daily Routine	22
Week 2: Eat a Healthy Breakfast and Less Processed Foods	24
Week 3: Exercise for a Mood Lift	27
Week 4: Devise a Diet Plan	29
Week 5 and Onwards: The Path to Consistency	32
Foods to Eat	35
Foods to Avoid	36
Sample Recipes	**38**
Carrot and Cashew Soup	39
Cucumber with Fennel and Creamy Avocado Dressing	41
Haddock Tacos	43
Arugula with Roasted Garlic Fig Dressing	46
Beets with Onions, Balsamic Vinegar, and Rosemary	48
Broccoli Salad	50
Vegetarian Egg Muffins	52
Lentil Soup	54
Spinach and Rice Haddock	56
Fish Steak	58
Tomato Basil and Tilapia	60
Spanish Rice	62
Instant Pot Broccoli	64

Baked Salmon	66
Grilled Chicken Breast	68
Conclusion	**70**
FAQ	**73**
References and Helpful Links	**76**

Introduction

In a world where diet trends ebb and flow with the seasons, a groundbreaking dietary strategy emerges. The Circadian Diet Guide offers more than just another trend; it presents a lifestyle adjustment deeply rooted in the science of our internal clocks. This innovative guide reveals a method of eating that aligns perfectly with your circadian rhythm, promising to revolutionize your approach to meal timing, nutrition, and overall well-being.

At the heart of the Circadian Diet lies the principle that our bodies operate on a 24-hour cycle, known as the circadian rhythm. This natural internal clock influences everything from our sleep cycles to hormone release and metabolism. By synchronizing your eating habits with this biological rhythm, the Circadian Diet Guide paves the way for improved metabolic health, enhanced sleep quality, and an overall increase in energy and vitality.

The guide meticulously unpacks the science of circadian rhythms, elucidating how different foods and their consumption times can significantly affect our bodies. It goes beyond simply listing foods to eat; it provides insights into the best times for consumption to ensure optimal fueling of your body when it's most receptive. This strategic approach to meal timing is crafted to bolster your body's natural functions, resulting in more efficient digestion, energy utilization, and, ultimately, effective weight management.

There's no longer a need to follow generic diet plans that disregard your body's unique rhythm. The Circadian Diet Guide offers a customized approach, featuring flexible eating windows and tailored food recommendations. Whether you are an early riser or prefer the night, the guide delivers actionable advice on adjusting your eating patterns to complement your circadian rhythm.

But the advantages extend beyond weight control. Adhering to a diet aligned with your circadian rhythm can also sharpen mental clarity, boost mood, and fortify the immune system. This comprehensive approach transcends mere weight loss, emphasizing holistic health and overall well-being.

In this guide, we will talk about the following:

- What is Circadian Rhythm?
- How Circadian Rhythm Affects Metabolism
- The Circadian Rhythm Diet
- How to Follow a Circadian Diet
- Foods to Eat and To Avoid

- Sample Recipes

Are you ready to bring your diet into harmony with your body's internal clock? The Circadian Diet Guide stands as your all-inclusive companion to making enlightened decisions about when and what to eat. Filled with straightforward meal plans, appetizing recipes, and practical tips, this guide is your key to integrating circadian eating effortlessly into your daily life.

Keep reading to learn more about how the Circadian Rhythm Diet can transform your health and well-being, and unlock the secrets to successfully implementing this revolutionary approach to eating. Remember, it's not just about weight loss - it's about achieving balance and optimal health through aligning with your body's natural rhythms. So let's dive in and discover what the Circadian Diet Guide has to offer!

What Is Circadian Rhythm?

The concept of Circadian Rhythm revolves around the 24-hour cycle of physiological processes that occur in every individual's body, governed by a "master clock" located in the brain. This master clock coordinates the schedules of various bodily functions by syncing with biological internal clocks present in each organ and body system, ensuring these functions occur at their optimal times throughout the day. Each of these biological clocks is dedicated to its specific area, producing circadian rhythms to keep everything running smoothly.

The National Sleep Foundation describes the circadian rhythm as an internal 24-hour clock that operates in the brain's background, alternating between periods of sleepiness and alertness at regular intervals, also known as our sleep/wake cycle.

Circadian rhythms are crucial for prompting the body to execute scheduled tasks efficiently, enhancing task performance through mechanisms like hormone secretion that regulates alertness or sleepiness, body temperature adjustment, and heart rate modulation. This explains why "morning people" naturally wake up early, and "night owls" tend to stay up late, as circadian rhythms strive to synchronize our physical activities with our internal body clock.

However, disruptions in these rhythms can occur due to modern lifestyles characterized by busy schedules, constant exposure to technology, irregular working hours, and continuous access to food, making it easy to ignore our natural bodily cues. When these disruptions happen, bodily functions may be forced to operate outside their scheduled times, leading to less efficient or effective performance.

Celebrity nutritionist, personal trainer, and author Harley Pasternak highlights the impact of sleep on our circadian rhythm, specifically focusing on two hormones, ghrelin and leptin, which regulate hunger. Ghrelin increases appetite, whereas leptin has the opposite effect. According to Pasternak, lack of sleep can disrupt our circadian rhythm, leading to increased levels of ghrelin and decreased levels of leptin, which in turn can cause heightened hunger and cravings for sugar.

How Circadian Rhythm Affects Metabolism

Metabolism is the process of breaking down food into smaller particles for the body to use. According to Dr. Milosavljevic, metabolism is not just about what happens inside your stomach. It may also refer to the biochemical processes happening. Something that has an impact on your metabolism that widely influences your health and whole wellbeing.

Cortisol is the hormone responsible for stimulating your body's metabolism. It is also known as the "get up and go" hormone or the stress hormone. Cortisol is triggered by our body's circadian rhythm. It supports metabolism and the functioning of your thyroid and provides the energy your body needs for you to fulfill your daily endeavors.

The Circadian Rhythm Diet

Our natural body clock and our external environment are synchronized through cues like the timing of our meals and exposure to sunlight. A circadian rhythm diet is a form of time-restricted eating plan where we eat in sync with this internal clock.

Dr. Milosavljevic stated that due to receiving a kick start brought by cortisol during metabolism, the food we consume has a higher possibility to be burned and converted as fuel, instead of being stored by our body as fat. Our body releases cortisol 2 times a day, the first one is released every early morning, and another one every late morning.

While the reverse is true every evening. Every time the sun sets, our body automatically feels the want to wind down and prepare for sleep. Our body responds to lower cortisol levels as part of the winding down. Consuming food late at night will most likely be stored by the body as fat since the cortisol level is decreasing. Circadian rhythm can help regulate how the calories are used by syncing up our time to eat early every morning and refrain from eating every early evening.

According to Dr. Milosavljevic, using the natural cycle of your body to shape your eating habits can greatly help in cutting off some pounds, and eating food from 7 AM to 7 PM is the ideal time for our body's needs. Knowing this, we are expected to say goodbye to eating our midnight snacks and get along with our body's cortisol peaks and circadian rhythm, maintaining a good diet that aligns with our body's "master clock".

Jessica Shand, a Naturopathic Nutrition Coach and the Founder of eatnourishandglow.com called the circadian diet the 'body clock diet'. According to her, the circadian diet is a time-restricted way of eating, working in sync with our body's internal body clock. She said that it would mean eating larger meals at the end of the day and making our last meal of the day lighter and smaller.

Anyone can benefit from this type of diet especially those who have metabolic problems and diseases like type 2 diabetes and obesity. According to dietitians, a circadian rhythm diet may also help those who are trying to cut down evening or late-night snacking and require some boundaries to help break the habit.

Just a reminder, you must speak to your dietitian or doctor first before kick-starting this new diet.

Principles of The Circadian Diet

The circadian diet is a novel approach to eating that emphasizes synchronizing your meal times with your body's natural circadian rhythms. This diet is rooted in the understanding that our bodies are designed to process food more efficiently at certain times of the day, based on our internal biological clock. Here are the key principles of the circadian diet:

1. ***Eat with the Sun***: One of the core tenets of the circadian diet is to eat in alignment with natural light patterns. This means consuming the majority of your calories during daylight hours, ideally when the sun is up. The rationale behind this principle is that our metabolism and digestive system are more active during these times, improving nutrient absorption and energy use.
2. ***Larger Meals Earlier***: The circadian diet advises having a hearty breakfast and lunch, followed by a lighter dinner. This pattern aligns with the body's natural rhythm of higher metabolic activity earlier in the day, which gradually decreases as the day progresses. By eating larger meals when your metabolism is at its peak, you support better digestion and energy distribution throughout the day.
3. ***Limited Eating Window***: Similar to intermittent fasting, the circadian diet recommends limiting your

eating window to a specific number of hours in the day—often around 8 to 12 hours. This encourages a fasting period when the sun is down, allowing your body to focus on rest and repair rather than digestion during the night.
4. *Avoid Late-Night Eating*: Eating late at night goes against your body's circadian rhythm, as it prepares for sleep. Late meals can disrupt sleep patterns and negatively impact digestion and metabolism. The circadian diet emphasizes finishing your last meal at least a couple of hours before bedtime to ensure your body is primed for restorative sleep.
5. *Consistency is Key*: Sticking to regular meal times helps reinforce your body's internal clock, making it easier to adhere to the circadian diet. Consistency in meal timing not only aids in better digestion and metabolism but also helps regulate hunger cues and reduces the likelihood of overeating.
6. *Focus on Nutrient-Dense Foods*: While the timing of meals is crucial in the circadian diet, the quality of food consumed is equally important. Prioritizing whole foods, rich in nutrients, supports overall health and aligns with the body's needs throughout the day. Including a variety of fruits, vegetables, whole grains, lean proteins, and healthy fats ensures you're getting a balanced diet within the eating patterns suggested by the circadian model.

By adhering to these principles, the circadian diet aims to optimize health by aligning eating patterns with the body's internal clock, thus improving metabolism, enhancing sleep quality, and supporting overall well-being.

The Benefits of the Circadian Rhythm Diet

The Circadian Rhythm diet, which aligns eating patterns with the body's natural circadian rhythms, offers a variety of benefits for overall health and well-being. Here are some of the key advantages of following this dietary approach:

1. *Improved Metabolism*: Eating in sync with your circadian rhythm can significantly optimize metabolic functions. By consuming meals at times when the body is naturally more prepared to digest and process food, individuals can enhance their metabolism.
2. *Weight Management*: This diet has been associated with weight loss. Aligning meal times with the body's internal clock helps in managing body weight more effectively.
3. *Enhanced Glucose Tolerance*: Following a circadian rhythm-based eating pattern improves glucose tolerance. This can be particularly beneficial for individuals with or at risk of developing diabetes.
4. *Protection Against Fatty Liver*: The diet plays a role in protecting against conditions such as fatty liver by

ensuring that food intake supports the body's natural processes.
5. ***Increased Metabolic Flexibility***: Adapting to a circadian rhythm diet increases the body's metabolic flexibility, enabling it to switch between burning carbohydrates and fats more efficiently.
6. ***Reduction in Problematic Blood Lipids***: Consuming meals according to circadian rhythms helps in reducing levels of problematic blood lipids, contributing to cardiovascular health.
7. ***Synchronization of Biological Rhythms***: Meal timing can synchronize the body's biological rhythms, including those governing metabolism and sleep, leading to improved health outcomes.
8. ***Reduced Inflammation***: Eating in alignment with your body's natural cycles can help reduce inflammation levels, enhancing overall health.
9. ***Optimized Hormonal Balance***: This dietary approach supports the timely release of hormones, maintaining a balance that benefits various bodily functions, including sleep and stress response.
10. ***Improved Digestive Health***: By eating by the body's circadian rhythms, individuals can experience enhancements in digestive efficiency and a reduction in gastrointestinal issues.
11. ***Better Sleep Quality***: Avoiding late-night eating as recommended by the circadian rhythm diet can lead to

improved sleep quality, as digestion does not interfere with the body's restorative processes.
12. ***Increased Energy Levels***: Properly timed meals can result in higher energy levels throughout the day, aligning with the body's natural activity periods.
13. ***Suitability for Metabolic Diseases***: Individuals with metabolic diseases, like obesity and type 2 diabetes, may find the circadian rhythm diet particularly beneficial for managing and improving their conditions.

The Circadian Rhythm diet, by promoting eating patterns that resonate with the body's natural timings, offers a holistic approach to improving health, supporting weight management, enhancing metabolic health, and contributing to overall well-being.

Disadvantages of The Circadian Diet

While the circadian diet, which harmonizes eating patterns with the body's natural circadian rhythms, has been widely lauded for its numerous health benefits, it's important to recognize that there are some potential disadvantages or challenges associated with this dietary approach. However, it is also crucial to note that for many individuals, the benefits significantly outweigh these disadvantages.

1. ***Adaptation Period***: Some individuals may find it challenging to adapt to the specific eating windows

recommended by the circadian diet, especially if their lifestyle or work schedule does not align neatly with typical daylight hours. This can lead to a period of adjustment where one might struggle with hunger pangs or low energy.

2. ***Social and Lifestyle Constraints***: Social events, family dinners, or professional obligations that involve food outside of the designated eating times can pose difficulties for those strictly following the circadian diet. This may require more planning and could potentially lead to feelings of isolation or missing out.
3. ***Reduced Flexibility***: For those who are used to snacking or eating at various times throughout the day, the circadian diet's emphasis on restricted eating windows can be perceived as less flexible, making it a difficult transition.
4. ***Potential Nutritional Imbalances***: Without careful planning, there's a risk that adherents might not get a balanced intake of nutrients if they significantly reduce their eating windows or unintentionally skip essential meals.

Though these challenges might seem daunting, there are ways to overcome them while still reaping the benefits of the circadian diet. One can start by gradually adjusting their eating windows, allowing for more flexibility in social situations or finding alternative options that fit within the designated eating times.

How to Follow a Circadian Diet

Now that we have discussed the benefits and potential challenges of the circadian diet, it's time to learn how to follow this eating pattern. Here are some tips for week 5:

Week 1: Assess your Daily Routine

This week, take some time to assess your daily routine and identify the times when you feel most hungry or have cravings for certain foods. This will help you determine the best eating windows for your body and lifestyle.

1. **Consider Reducing your "Eating Window"**

    It might seem impossible for you to eat within an 8-hour window most especially when you have a family to take care of, or have a shift work type of job, or when you simply consider yourself as a person who avoids feeling hungry. Everybody faces various challenges within his or her schedule, and because of this, experts suggest starting a circadian diet through mindfulness about the time you eat.

"Eating window" is the number of hours between your first and last meal of each day. Some research studies suggest that reducing the window from 14 hours to 10 hours or even less will result in a metabolic benefit.

A team from the Salk Institute for Biological Studies suggests beginning with a 12-hour eating window and working the way up until the ideal 8-hour period, when weight loss, prediabetic reversal, and endurance might occur within two months. They refer to it as the "magic time". They also suggest that the duration might also result in the end of period pains, panic attacks, and premenopausal migraines.

2. **Start with a Simple Morning Adjustment**

It might sound like an impossible stretch for most people doing a 14 to 16-hour "cleansing" phase of eating nothing between breakfast and dinner, however, according to dietitians, much of it depends on perception. Dietitians say that after almost 2 to 3 weeks, people will recognize that things their body wants are merely out of habit, like brushing their teeth two to three times a day.

Tiny changes to your regular morning routine will surely result in a huge difference. For example, instead of eating right after you wake up, consider taking your breakfast to work, and as usual, at night eating with your family. People who rest at 6:00 P.M. or 7 P.M. are less likely to indulge in alcohol and dessert and will consequently realize and see the big difference in their health.

3. **Give Yourself a Week to Adjust**

According to a dietitian, the first week will be very difficult. You will feel hunger, but it is a healthy hunger. After almost three to four hours of eating nothing, the body is deprived of sugar and it is ready to tap into the carbohydrates that are stored in your liver, which is a good thing.

Overnight fasting is a very different story: Every morning, in the last four hours of fasting, you are burning fats. Fat then is converted to good ketone bodies because it fuels your heart and brain. But this does not mean skipping meals. It is about closing the window, so you are not eating during the times that your body does not need fuel.

Week 2: Eat a Healthy Breakfast and Less Processed Foods

In the second week, it is important to focus on eating a healthy breakfast and reducing processed foods in your diet.

This means opting for whole, unprocessed foods such as fruits, vegetables, whole grains, and lean protein sources.

Why Focus on a Healthy Breakfast?

Breakfast is often described as the most important meal of the day, and for a good reason, especially within the context of the circadian diet. Starting your day with a meal rich in nutrients can jumpstart your metabolism, aligning your body's energy use with its natural peak in the morning.

Dietitians recommend incorporating a balance of good fats, proteins, and fibers into your breakfast. Such a meal not only provides sustained energy but also helps keep hunger at bay, preventing the mid-morning slump and the temptation to snack on less healthy options.

Foods rich in healthy fats like avocados, nuts, and seeds, alongside high-fiber options such as whole grains and legumes, play a significant role in this meal. They work together to provide a sense of fullness and satisfaction. Proteins, from both plant and animal sources, are essential as well, aiding in muscle repair and growth while also contributing to satiety.

Less Processed Foods, More Whole Foods

The circadian diet also advocates for a reduction in the consumption of processed foods. These are often high in added sugars, unhealthy fats, and artificial ingredients, which can disrupt metabolic processes and lead to weight gain, among other health issues.

Instead, the focus should be on whole foods. These are foods in their natural or minimally processed state, which contain a plethora of vitamins, minerals, and other nutrients essential for optimal health.

For lunch, which should ideally be lighter than breakfast but still nutritious, aim for a balanced mix of healthy carbohydrates (like quinoa or sweet potatoes), proteins (such as grilled chicken or lentils), and fats (like olive oil or nuts). This combination supports your energy levels throughout the afternoon and prepares your body for the fasting period to come.

The 14-Hour Fast

Integrating a 14-hour fast into your daily routine is another key component of the circadian diet. This fasting period, which includes the time spent sleeping, allows your digestive system to rest and recuperate, potentially improving metabolic health and optimizing fat burning. It's suggested to begin this fasting window after an early dinner, refraining from late-night snacking to ensure the fast is uninterrupted.

In essence, adopting a circadian diet by focusing on a nutrient-rich breakfast and less processed foods, paired with mindful eating schedules, can be a powerful strategy for aligning our dietary habits with our body's natural rhythms.

This alignment has the potential to enhance overall health, energy levels, and perhaps even longevity.

Week 3: Exercise for a Mood Lift

In the third week of adopting a circadian diet, the focus shifts towards integrating exercise into your routine as a means to enhance mood and further align with your body's natural rhythms. Understanding the optimal times for physical activity can significantly amplify the benefits you receive, not just physically but also mentally and emotionally.

Morning Exercise Benefits

Exercising in the morning has been shown to kickstart your day in the best possible way. Engaging in outdoor activities or even workouts by a window allows for exposure to natural light, which has a profound impact on mood regulation.

According to sources like Johns Hopkins Medicine, natural light serves as a natural antidepressant by boosting serotonin levels, a neurotransmitter associated with feelings of well-being and happiness. This is particularly beneficial in the morning when the body's cortisol levels are naturally higher, helping to increase alertness and energy.

Furthermore, replacing your morning caffeine with a workout could be advantageous. Physical activity increases oxygen flow throughout the body and brain, enhancing cognitive function and overall vitality. It's a healthy, stimulating start that prepares you for the day ahead, potentially reducing reliance on stimulants like coffee.

Afternoon and Evening Exercise Advantages

For those looking to improve joint flexibility and muscle tone, scheduling workouts between 5:00 P.M. and 7:00 P.M. might be most beneficial. During this time, the body's temperature is naturally higher, making muscles more flexible and reducing the risk of injuries. This period is also when muscle strength and function peak, according to research shared by the National Center for Biotechnology Information (NCBI), making exercises more effective and potentially leading to better performance and results.

Additionally, engaging in physical activities in the late afternoon or early evening can serve as a fantastic way to decompress and relieve the stresses accumulated throughout the day. It provides a healthy outlet for releasing tension and can help ensure a sense of calm and relaxation in the evening, setting the stage for a good night's sleep.

Harmonizing Exercise with Circadian Rhythms

Aligning your exercise routine with your circadian rhythms is about more than just physical health; it's about creating a holistic balance that supports your mental and emotional well-being. By exercising outdoors in the morning, you're not only giving your body a boost of natural energy but also improving your mood and mental clarity, thanks to increased light exposure and enhanced oxygen flow. Meanwhile, opting for later workouts can maximize your physical potential and aid in stress relief.

Incorporating these practices into your circadian diet plan enhances the diet's effectiveness by not only focusing on what and when you eat but also on optimizing other aspects of your lifestyle to work in harmony with your body's natural cycles. This holistic approach can lead to improved health outcomes, greater well-being, and a more balanced and fulfilling life.

Week 4: Devise a Diet Plan

This week, we'll be focusing on creating a diet plan that works in harmony with your circadian rhythms and supports your overall well-being.

1. **Morning Rituals:**

   Hydration Upon Awakening: Start your day by drinking 16-32 ounces of warm water immediately after waking up to rehydrate your body, boost energy, and reduce inflammation. Optionally, add lemon to stimulate your liver. Wait 20-30 minutes before consuming breakfast.

2. **Breakfast Guidelines:**

   Protein-Rich Breakfast: Within an hour of waking, have a breakfast high in protein. Integrate vegetables into this meal and avoid simple or refined sugars and carbs. Calcium intake through yogurt is not recommended during morning hours. Pair your meal with caffeine only after finishing at least half of your breakfast, even though the morning isn't the optimal time for caffeine absorption.

3. Snacking Smart:

Mid-Morning Snack: Opt for a combination of vegetables and proteins for a nutritious snack.

4. Lunchtime Choices:

Balanced Lunch: For lunch, focus on a mix of vegetables and proteins, steering clear of sugars. You can include whole grains and complex carbohydrates like quinoa, brown rice, amaranth, and millet, but in moderation.

5. Afternoon Indulgences:

Afternoon Snack & Dessert: The mid-afternoon period is ideal for consuming sweets and fruits—eat fruits by themselves. It's also when the body best processes caffeine; however, to ensure quality sleep, it's advisable to limit caffeine consumption.

Desserts are better enjoyed before dinner, as this timing supports magnesium and calcium absorption. If you're not lactose intolerant, enjoy dairy products; otherwise, opt for greens, fish, or supplements for your calcium and magnesium intake, which are crucial for sleep and muscle relaxation.

6. **Dinner Dynamics:**

Nutritious Dinner: Dinner should consist of vegetables, light proteins, and complex carbohydrates like whole grains, yams, and sweet potatoes. These aid in blood sugar regulation, metabolism, and sleep quality. The evening is also the most suitable time for alcohol consumption.

7. **Hydration Habits:**

Fluid Intake: Maintaining hydration throughout the day is vital for diluting digestive juices and optimizing nutrient absorption from foods. Keeping a glass of water by your bed to drink upon waking at night is beneficial.

8. **Prioritizing Sleep:**

Quality Sleep for Health: Achieving good sleep is essential for glowing skin and gut health. During 14 hours of cleansing and deep sleep, the brain generates growth hormones that repair the skin and gut lining, renewing the skin layer every 10-15 days. Good sleep strengthens the immune system by enhancing the skin and gut barrier against viruses. Minimize caffeine intake in the afternoon and turn off electronic devices at least 30 minutes before bed. Consider calming music at night to facilitate peaceful sleep.

Week 5 and Onwards: The Path to Consistency

As you transition into Week 5 and beyond, the key to unlocking the full potential of your body's health lies in consistency. Establishing and maintaining a daily routine that aligns with your circadian rhythm is more than a habit—it's a lifestyle commitment that nurtures your physical, mental, and emotional well-being.

1. **The Power of Routine**

    Regular sleeping and eating habits serve as the foundation for optimizing your body's circadian rhythm. This internal clock governs countless biological processes, from metabolism to hormone release, significantly influencing your energy levels, mood, and overall health. By adhering to consistent routines, you provide your body with a predictable environment, enhancing its ability to function at its peak.

2. **Eating Patterns**

    A structured eating schedule trains your digestive system to anticipate meals, optimizing digestion and nutrient absorption. Consistency in meal timing helps regulate hunger hormones like ghrelin and leptin, reducing cravings and overeating. Commit to your meal and snack times, aligning them with natural daylight hours to support your metabolism and encourage efficient energy use.

3. **Sleep Hygiene**

   Equally crucial is a consistent sleep schedule. Aim for 7-9 hours of quality sleep nightly, going to bed, and waking up at the same times each day, even on weekends. This regularity reinforces your natural sleep-wake cycle, improving sleep quality and making it easier to fall asleep and wake up refreshed.

4. **Hydration and Exercise**

   Maintain hydration throughout the day, starting with warm water in the morning and continuing with regular fluid intake. Regular physical activity should also be a non-negotiable part of your routine. Exercise not only boosts mood and energy but also helps anchor your circadian rhythm, especially if done consistently at the same time each day.

5. **Mindfulness and Screen Time**

   Be mindful of electronic device use, particularly in the evening. Limiting screen time before bed supports melatonin production, essential for restful sleep.

Incorporate relaxation techniques such as meditation, reading, or gentle stretching into your nighttime routine to signal to your body that it's time to wind down.

6. **The Journey of Adaptation**

   Remember, establishing a new routine may require time and adjustment. Listen to your body and make modifications as needed to find what best supports your circadian rhythm. It's normal to encounter setbacks, but the key is perseverance and a willingness to adapt.

7. **Building on Progress**

   Celebrate the victories, no matter how small, and continue to build on the progress you've made. Over time, these practices will become second nature, significantly contributing to enhanced health, vitality, and happiness.

By committing to consistency in your daily routine and diet, you're investing in a future where your body operates harmoniously within the natural cycles it was designed to follow. Herein lies the secret to living a balanced, healthy life—today, tomorrow, and well into the future.

Foods to Eat

In the Circadian Diet, aligning your eating habits with your body's natural circadian rhythms can significantly enhance your health and well-being. The diet emphasizes the timing of your meals in addition to encouraging the consumption of specific types of foods. Here are key food groups and items that are particularly compatible with the Circadian Diet:

- *Whole Grains*: Opt for whole grains like oats, quinoa, brown rice, and whole wheat. These provide sustained energy and are rich in fiber, which helps keep you full and supports digestive health.
- *Lean Proteins*: Incorporate sources of lean protein such as poultry, fish, tofu, legumes, and eggs. Protein is essential for muscle repair, growth, and overall body function.
- *Healthy Fats*: Focus on healthy fats found in avocados, nuts, seeds, and olive oil. These fats are crucial for brain health, hormone production, and managing inflammation.
- *Fruits and Vegetables*: A wide variety of fruits and vegetables ensures a high intake of vitamins, minerals, antioxidants, and fiber. These nutrients support immune function, reduce disease risk, and promote overall health.
- *Fermented Foods*: Include fermented foods like yogurt, kefir, sauerkraut, and kombucha in your diet.

These are great for gut health, providing probiotics that help maintain a healthy digestive system.
- *Hydration*: While not a food, proper hydration is crucial. Drink plenty of water throughout the day, and you can also include herbal teas and other non-caffeinated, sugar-free beverages.
- *Nutrient-Dense Snacks*: If you need snacks, go for options that are rich in nutrients—think almond butter on whole-grain toast, fresh fruit, or a handful of nuts.

By focusing on these food groups and ensuring that you eat in harmony with your circadian rhythm, you can optimize your diet for better health and vitality.

Foods to Avoid

In the context of a Circadian Diet, where the timing and quality of your food intake are aligned with your body's natural circadian rhythms to optimize health, certain foods are generally recommended to be limited or avoided. These include:

- *Highly Processed Foods*: These are often high in added sugars, unhealthy fats, and artificial ingredients that can disrupt your body's natural processes and negatively impact metabolic health.
- *Sugar-Sweetened Beverages*: Drinks that are high in sugar can lead to spikes in blood sugar levels and can

disrupt your natural eating patterns, contributing to weight gain and other health issues.

- ***Heavy Meals Late at Night***: Consuming large, heavy meals close to bedtime can disrupt your sleep cycle and hinder the natural fasting period your body undergoes overnight, impacting overall circadian alignment.
- ***Caffeinated Beverages Late in the Day***: Caffeine can interfere with your ability to fall asleep if consumed late in the day, disrupting your natural sleep-wake cycle and, consequently, your eating schedule aligned with circadian rhythms.
- ***Alcohol***: Drinking alcohol, especially in the evening, can affect your sleep quality and duration, which in turn can disturb your circadian rhythm and negatively impact your dietary habits.
- ***Refined Carbohydrates and Sugary Snacks***: Foods high in refined sugars and carbohydrates can cause rapid spikes and drops in blood sugar levels, potentially leading to energy crashes and cravings that disrupt eating patterns aligned with your circadian clock.

By focusing on whole, nutrient-dense foods and avoiding these types of foods, you can better align your diet with your circadian rhythms, supporting optimal health, metabolism, and well-being.

Sample Recipes

When it comes to eating for optimal circadian health, whole and unprocessed foods are always the best option. Here are a few sample recipes to help get you started:

Carrot and Cashew Soup

Ingredients:

- 1 tablespoon extra virgin olive oil
- 3/4 cup cashews, soaked for at least 4 hours, then drained and rinsed
- 1 large onion, chopped
- 2 cloves garlic, chopped
- 500 grams / 1 lb of carrots, peeled and sliced into coins
- 1/2 inch fresh ginger, grated
- 6 cups vegetable broth (ensure it's low sodium for a healthier option)
- Salt to taste (optional)
- Freshly ground black pepper to taste
- A touch of coconut milk for serving (optional, adds creaminess)
- Fresh herbs like parsley or cilantro for garnish

Instructions:

1. Prepare the Base: In a large pot, heat the extra virgin olive oil over medium heat. Add the chopped onion and garlic, sautéing until they become translucent and fragrant, about 5 minutes.
2. Add Carrots and Spices: Add the sliced carrots and grated ginger to the pot. Cook for another 5-7 minutes, stirring occasionally, allowing the carrots to soften slightly and the flavors to meld.

3. Integrate Cashews: Pour in the soaked and rinsed cashews along with the vegetable broth. Bring the mixture to a boil, then reduce the heat to allow it to simmer. Cover the pot and let it cook until the carrots are fully tender, about 20-30 minutes.
4. Blend to Perfection: Once the carrots are tender, use an immersion blender directly in the pot to blend the soup until smooth and creamy. Alternatively, you can carefully transfer the soup in batches to a blender to achieve the same result. Ensure the soup is completely smooth.
5. Final Seasoning: Taste the soup and adjust the seasoning with salt and freshly ground black pepper as needed. For a touch of creaminess, you can stir in a bit of coconut milk at this stage.
6. Serve Warm: Serve the soup warm, garnished with a sprinkle of fresh herbs like parsley or cilantro. For an added touch of texture, you could top each serving with a few whole or chopped cashews.

Cucumber with Fennel and Creamy Avocado Dressing

Ingredients:

For the Salad:

- 2 large cucumbers, thinly sliced
- 1 fennel bulb, thinly sliced
- 1/2 red onion, thinly sliced
- A handful of fresh dill, roughly chopped
- Salt (optional) and freshly ground black pepper to taste

For the Creamy Avocado Dressing:

- 1 ripe avocado
- 1/4 cup extra virgin olive oil
- Juice of 1 lemon
- 1 clove garlic
- Salt (optional) to taste
- Water, as needed to adjust consistency

Instructions:

1. Prepare the Salad Base: In a large mixing bowl, combine the thinly sliced cucumbers, fennel bulb, and red onion. Add the roughly chopped fresh dill, and gently toss to mix the ingredients.
2. Make the Creamy Avocado Dressing: In a blender, combine the ripe avocado, extra virgin olive oil, lemon juice, and garlic. Blend until smooth. If the dressing is

too thick, add a small amount of water to reach a creamy, pourable consistency. Season with salt to taste, if desired.

3. **Combine and Serve:** Drizzle the creamy avocado dressing over the salad mixture. Toss gently to ensure that the cucumber, fennel, and onion slices are evenly coated with the dressing. Taste and adjust seasoning with salt (if using) and freshly ground black pepper.
4. **Chill and Enjoy:** For the best flavor, allow the salad to chill in the refrigerator for about 30 minutes before serving. This step helps the flavors meld together and enhances the refreshing quality of the salad.

Haddock Tacos

Ingredients:

For the Fish:

- 4 haddock filets (about 6 ounces each), skin removed
- Juice of 1 lime
- 1 tablespoon olive oil
- 1 teaspoon ground cumin
- 1 teaspoon smoked paprika
- Salt (optional) and freshly ground black pepper to taste

For the Slaw:

- 1/2 small red cabbage, thinly sliced
- 1 carrot, julienned or grated
- 1/4 cup fresh cilantro, chopped
- Juice of 1 lime
- Salt (optional) and freshly ground black pepper to taste

For the Avocado Cream:

- 1 ripe avocado
- 1/4 cup Greek yogurt (use a dairy-free alternative if necessary)
- Juice of 1/2 lime
- Salt (optional) to taste

Additional:

- Whole-grain tortillas or corn tortillas

- Additional lime wedges for serving

Instructions:

1. Marinate the Fish: Place the haddock filets in a shallow dish. Mix lime juice, olive oil, ground cumin, smoked paprika, salt (if using), and black pepper in a small bowl. Pour the marinade over the fish, ensuring each piece is well-coated. Cover and refrigerate for at least 30 minutes.
2. Prepare the Slaw: In a large bowl, combine red cabbage, carrot, and cilantro. Toss with lime juice, salt (if using), and black pepper. Set aside to allow the flavors to meld.
3. Make the Avocado Cream: Blend the ripe avocado, Greek yogurt, lime juice, and salt (if using) in a blender or food processor until smooth. Adjust the seasoning as needed.
4. Cook the Fish: Heat a non-stick skillet over medium heat. Add the marinated haddock filets and cook for 3-4 minutes on each side, or until the fish is opaque and flakes easily. Remove from heat and break the fish into smaller pieces with a fork.
5. Assemble the Tacos: Warm the tortillas according to package instructions. Place a scoop of the slaw on each tortilla, add pieces of cooked haddock on top, and drizzle with avocado cream.

6. Serve: Arrange the tacos on plates, serving with additional lime wedges on the side for squeezing over the tacos.

Arugula with Roasted Garlic Fig Dressing

Ingredients:

For the Salad:

- 4 cups fresh arugula, washed and dried
- 1/2 cup thinly sliced red onion
- 1/2 cup pecans, toasted and roughly chopped
- 1 cup fresh figs, quartered
- Optional: goat cheese crumbles for topping

For the Roasted Garlic Fig Dressing:

- 1 head of garlic, roasted
- 3 tablespoons fig preserves
- 2 tablespoons apple cider vinegar
- 1 tablespoon Dijon mustard
- 1/4 cup extra virgin olive oil
- Salt (optional) and freshly ground black pepper to taste

Instructions:

1. Roast the Garlic: Preheat your oven to 400°F (200°C). Cut the top off the head of garlic to expose the cloves. Drizzle with a little olive oil, wrap in aluminum foil, and roast in the oven for about 30-35 minutes, or until tender and golden. Allow to cool, then squeeze out the garlic cloves.
2. Prepare the Dressing: In a blender, combine the roasted garlic cloves, fig preserves, apple cider vinegar, and

Dijon mustard. Blend until smooth. While blending, slowly add in the olive oil until the dressing is emulsified. Season with salt (if using) and freshly ground black pepper to taste. Adjust the consistency with a little water if necessary.
3. Assemble the Salad: In a large salad bowl, combine the arugula, red onion, and toasted pecans. Add the fresh figs on top and toss lightly to combine.
4. Dress and Serve: Drizzle the roasted garlic fig dressing over the salad just before serving. Gently toss to ensure all ingredients are well-coated. For an added touch of luxury, top with goat cheese crumbles if desired.
5. Enjoy: Serve this delightful salad as a standalone meal for lunch or as an elegant side dish for an early dinner, aligning with the Circadian Rhythm diet's recommendation for lighter, plant-based meals earlier in the day.

Beets with Onions, Balsamic Vinegar, and Rosemary

Ingredients:

- 4 medium-sized beets, peeled and cut into wedges
- 1 large red onion, sliced into wedges
- 3 tablespoons extra virgin olive oil
- 2 tablespoons balsamic vinegar
- 2 teaspoons fresh rosemary, finely chopped
- Salt (optional) and freshly ground black pepper to taste

Instructions:

1. Preheat Oven: Start by preheating your oven to 375°F (190°C). This moderate temperature allows the beets and onions to roast slowly, caramelizing their natural sugars.
2. Prepare the Beets and Onions: In a large mixing bowl, toss the beet wedges and red onion wedges with the extra virgin olive oil until they are well coated. Sprinkle the fresh rosemary over the top and season with salt (if using) and freshly ground black pepper. Mix well to ensure all pieces are evenly seasoned.
3. Roast: Spread the beet and onion mixture in a single layer on a baking sheet lined with parchment paper or lightly greased with olive oil. Roast in the preheated oven for 35-40 minutes, or until the beets are tender and the edges of the onions start to brown. Halfway

through the roasting time, drizzle the balsamic vinegar over the vegetables and give them a gentle stir to ensure even flavoring.
4. Serve Warm: Once roasted to perfection, remove the beets and onions from the oven and allow them to cool slightly. They are best served warm, allowing the flavors of the balsamic vinegar and rosemary to shine through.
5. Finishing Touches: If desired, garnish with a sprinkle of additional fresh rosemary before serving for an added burst of flavor and color.

Broccoli Salad

Ingredients:

For the Salad:

- 4 cups of fresh broccoli florets (approximately 2 medium heads of broccoli)
- 1/2 cup red onion, finely chopped
- 1/2 cup almonds, sliced or chopped (for added crunch)
- 1/2 cup dried cranberries or raisins (ensure no added sugar for strict diet adherence)
- Optional: 1/4 cup sunflower seeds or pumpkin seeds for extra texture

For the Dressing:

- 1/3 cup apple cider vinegar
- 2 tablespoons extra virgin olive oil
- 1 tablespoon Dijon mustard
- 1 tablespoon honey (use a natural sweetener alternative if honey is restricted)
- Salt (optional) and freshly ground black pepper to taste

Instructions:

1. Prepare the Broccoli: Wash the broccoli florets and dry them thoroughly. Chop the florets into bite-sized pieces if needed. For a softer texture, you can blanch the broccoli florets for 1-2 minutes in boiling water, then immediately rinse under cold water and drain.

2. Mix Salad Ingredients: In a large salad bowl, combine the chopped broccoli, red onion, almonds, and dried cranberries or raisins. If using, add the sunflower seeds or pumpkin seeds as well.
3. Make the Dressing: In a small bowl, whisk together the apple cider vinegar, extra virgin olive oil, Dijon mustard, and honey until well combined. Season with salt (if using) and freshly ground black pepper to taste.
4. Combine and Chill: Pour the dressing over the salad and toss well to ensure all the ingredients are evenly coated. For the best flavor, cover and refrigerate the salad for at least one hour before serving to allow the flavors to meld together.
5. Serve: Serve the chilled broccoli salad as a refreshing and nutritious side dish or as a standalone meal for lunch. The vibrant colors and diverse textures make this salad not only pleasing to the palate but also to the eye.

Vegetarian Egg Muffins

Ingredients:

- 8 large eggs
- 1/2 cup milk (use almond milk or another non-dairy milk for a dairy-free version)
- 1 cup spinach, finely chopped
- 1/2 cup bell peppers, diced (any color)
- 1/4 cup onions, finely chopped
- 1/2 cup mushrooms, diced
- 1/2 cup cherry tomatoes, quartered
- 1/4 cup feta cheese, crumbled (omit for a dairy-free version)
- Salt (optional) and freshly ground black pepper to taste
- Non-stick cooking spray or olive oil for greasing

Instructions:

1. Preheat Oven: Begin by preheating your oven to 375°F (190°C). This ensures the muffins cook evenly and obtain a golden color.
2. Prepare the Vegetables: Wash and finely chop the spinach, bell peppers, onions, mushrooms, and cherry tomatoes. The small size allows them to cook quickly and distribute evenly among the egg muffins.
3. Mix Eggs: In a large bowl, whisk the eggs and milk together until well combined. Season with salt (if using) and freshly ground black pepper.

4. Add Vegetables and Cheese: Stir in the chopped vegetables and crumbled feta cheese into the egg mixture. Feta cheese adds a nice tangy flavor, but it can be omitted if you're avoiding dairy.
5. Grease Muffin Tin: Lightly grease a 12-cup muffin tin with non-stick cooking spray or olive oil to prevent sticking.
6. Fill Muffin Cups: Evenly divide the egg and vegetable mixture among the muffin cups. Each cup should be filled approximately 3/4 of the way to allow room for the muffins to rise as they bake.
7. Bake: Place the muffin tin in the preheated oven and bake for 20-25 minutes, or until the muffins are set in the middle and lightly golden on top.
8. Cool and Serve: Allow the muffins to cool in the pan for a few minutes before transferring them to a wire rack to cool completely. Serve warm or at room temperature.

Lentil Soup

Ingredients:

- 1 cup dried lentils (green, brown, or red), rinsed and drained
- 2 tablespoons olive oil
- 1 onion, diced
- 2 garlic cloves, minced
- 2 carrots, peeled and diced
- 2 celery stalks, diced
- 1 small zucchini, diced (optional)
- 1 teaspoon ground cumin
- 1/2 teaspoon smoked paprika
- 4 cups vegetable broth (or water)
- 1 can (14 oz) diced tomatoes, with their juice
- Salt (optional) and freshly ground black pepper to taste
- 2 cups spinach leaves, roughly chopped
- Juice of 1 lemon

Instructions:

1. Sauté Vegetables: In a large pot, heat the olive oil over medium heat. Add the diced onion and sauté until translucent, about 3-5 minutes. Add the minced garlic, carrots, celery, and zucchini (if using), and continue to sauté for another 5 minutes until the vegetables are slightly softened.

2. Add Spices: Stir in the ground cumin and smoked paprika, cooking for one minute until fragrant.
3. Cook Lentils: Add the rinsed lentils to the pot along with the vegetable broth (or water) and diced tomatoes with their juice. Season with salt (if using) and freshly ground black pepper. Bring the mixture to a boil, then reduce the heat to low, cover, and simmer for 25-30 minutes, or until the lentils are tender.
4. Finish Soup: Once the lentils are cooked, stir in the chopped spinach and cook until wilted about 2-3 minutes. Remove the soup from the heat and stir in the lemon juice.
5. Serve: Taste and adjust the seasoning as needed. Serve the soup warm in bowls, optionally garnishing with fresh herbs like parsley or cilantro for an added burst of flavor.

Spinach and Rice Haddock

Ingredients:

- 4 haddock filets (about 6 ounces each)
- 2 cups cooked brown rice
- 4 cups fresh spinach, roughly chopped
- 2 tablespoons olive oil
- Juice of 1 lemon
- 2 garlic cloves, minced
- 1 teaspoon dried oregano
- Salt (optional) and freshly ground black pepper to taste
- Lemon slices for garnish

Instructions:

1. Preheat Oven: Start by preheating your oven to 375°F (190°C). This will ensure that the haddock cooks through evenly without drying out.
2. Prepare the Spinach Rice: In a large skillet, heat 1 tablespoon of olive oil over medium heat. Add the minced garlic and sauté for about 1 minute until fragrant. Add the fresh spinach and cook until slightly wilted, about 2-3 minutes. Stir in the cooked brown rice, half of the lemon juice, dried oregano, salt (if using), and black pepper. Mix well until all ingredients are combined and heated through. Remove from heat and set aside.

3. Bake the Haddock: Place the haddock filets in a single layer in a baking dish lightly greased with olive oil. Drizzle the remaining tablespoon of olive oil and the rest of the lemon juice over the filets. Season with salt (if using) and freshly ground black pepper. Bake in the preheated oven for 12-15 minutes or until the fish flakes easily with a fork.
4. Serve: Divide the spinach and rice mixture among plates. Carefully place a baked haddock filet on top of each bed of spinach rice. Garnish with lemon slices.

Fish Steak

Ingredients:

- 4 fish steaks (cod, halibut, salmon, or any other preferred lean fish), about 6 ounces each
- 2 tablespoons olive oil
- Juice of 1 lemon
- 2 garlic cloves, minced
- 1 teaspoon dried thyme
- Salt (optional) and freshly ground black pepper to taste
- Lemon slices and fresh dill for garnish

Instructions:

1. Marinate the Fish: Combine olive oil, lemon juice, minced garlic, dried thyme, a pinch of salt (optional), and black pepper in a small bowl. Put the fish steaks in a shallow container and drizzle the prepared marinade over them, ensuring each side is evenly covered. Cover and refrigerate for at least 30 minutes to allow the flavors to infuse.
2. Preheat the Grill or Pan: If you're grilling, preheat your grill to medium-high heat. If you're using a stovetop, heat a grill pan over medium-high heat.
3. Cook the Fish Steaks: Remove the fish steaks from the marinade, letting any excess drip off. Place the fish on the grill or in the pan. Cook for about 4-5 minutes on each side, or until the fish is opaque throughout and

flakes easily with a fork. The actual cooking time may vary depending on the thickness of the fish steaks.
4. Serve: Transfer the cooked fish steaks to plates. Garnish with lemon slices and fresh dill. Serve immediately.

Tomato Basil and Tilapia

Ingredients:

- 4 tilapia filets (about 6 ounces each)
- 2 tablespoons olive oil
- 3 ripe tomatoes, diced
- 2 garlic cloves, minced
- 1/4 cup fresh basil leaves, chopped
- Juice of 1 lemon
- Salt (optional) and freshly ground black pepper to taste
- Additional fresh basil leaves for garnish

Instructions:

1. Preheat Oven: Begin by preheating your oven to 375°F (190°C). This gentle cooking method preserves the delicate flavor of the tilapia while ensuring it cooks through evenly.
2. Prepare the Tomato Basil Mixture: In a medium bowl, mix the diced tomatoes, minced garlic, chopped basil, lemon juice, salt (if using), and freshly ground black pepper. Set aside to allow the flavors to meld while you prepare the fish.
3. Prepare Tilapia: Place the tilapia filets in a single layer in a baking dish. Drizzle with 1 tablespoon of olive oil and season with a little salt (if using) and black pepper.

4. Top with Tomato Basil Mixture: Spoon the tomato basil mixture evenly over the tilapia filets, ensuring they are well covered.
5. Bake: Place the baking dish in the preheated oven and bake for 15-20 minutes, or until the tilapia flakes easily with a fork and the tomatoes are soft and slightly caramelized.
6. Serve: Remove the baking dish from the oven. Carefully transfer the tilapia filets onto plates, spooning any of the tomato basil mixture and juices left in the dish over the top. Garnish with additional fresh basil leaves.

Spanish Rice

Ingredients:

- 1 cup brown rice, rinsed
- 2 tablespoons olive oil
- 1 onion, finely chopped
- 2 garlic cloves, minced
- 1 bell pepper (any color), diced
- 1 can (14 oz) diced tomatoes, with their juice
- 2 cups vegetable broth (or water)
- 1 teaspoon smoked paprika
- 1 teaspoon ground cumin
- Salt (optional) and freshly ground black pepper to taste
- Fresh cilantro, chopped (for garnish)
- Juice of 1 lime

Instructions:

1. Cook the Rice: Start by cooking the brown rice according to package instructions, using water or vegetable broth for added flavor. Once cooked, set aside.
2. Sauté Veggies: Heat the olive oil in a large skillet over medium heat. Add the chopped onion and sauté until translucent, about 5 minutes. Add the minced garlic and diced bell pepper, cooking for another 3-4 minutes until the pepper is tender.

3. Add Tomatoes and Spices: Stir in the diced tomatoes (with their juice), smoked paprika, and ground cumin. Cook for about 5 minutes, allowing the flavors to meld together. Season with salt (if using) and freshly ground black pepper to taste.
4. Combine Rice: Add the cooked brown rice to the skillet, mixing well to ensure it's fully integrated with the vegetables and spice mixture. Cook for an additional 5 minutes, stirring occasionally, to allow the rice to absorb the flavors and the liquid to reduce slightly.
5. Finish and Serve: Remove the skillet from the heat. Squeeze the juice of one lime over the rice and mix well. Taste and adjust seasoning as needed. Garnish with fresh chopped cilantro before serving.

Instant Pot Broccoli

Ingredients:

- 1 large head of broccoli
- 1 cup water
- 1 tablespoon olive oil
- Juice of 1/2 lemon
- Salt (optional) and freshly ground black pepper to taste

Instructions:

1. Prepare the Broccoli: Start by washing the head of broccoli. Then, cut the broccoli into florets of uniform size to ensure even cooking. You can also trim and use the stems if you like, just peel them and slice them thinly.
2. Add Water to the Instant Pot: Pour 1 cup of water into the bottom of your Instant Pot. This will create the steam needed to cook the broccoli.
3. Place the Broccoli in the Instant Pot: Insert the steaming basket or trivet into the Instant Pot. Then, place the broccoli florets on top of the basket or trivet. Drizzling the olive oil and lemon juice over the broccoli before cooking can help add flavor.
4. Cook the Broccoli: Secure the lid of your Instant Pot and set the valve to the "Sealing" position. Use the manual setting to cook on high pressure for 0 minutes. Yes, 0 minutes is correct—the broccoli cooks to

perfection simply with the time it takes to come up to pressure.
5. Quick Release and Season: Once the Instant Pot has finished cooking, carefully do a quick release by moving the valve to the "Venting" position. Once all the steam has been released and the pin drops, safely open the lid. Transfer the broccoli to a serving dish, season with salt (if using) and freshly ground black pepper, and toss gently to combine.

Baked Salmon

Ingredients:

- 4 salmon filets (about 6 ounces each)
- 2 tablespoons olive oil
- 1 lemon, thinly sliced
- 2 garlic cloves, minced
- 1 teaspoon dried dill or fresh dill to taste
- Salt (optional) and freshly ground black pepper to taste
- Fresh parsley, chopped (for garnish)

Instructions:

1. Preheat Oven: Begin by preheating your oven to 400°F (200°C). This temperature ensures the salmon will cook through evenly while retaining its moisture and tenderness.
2. Prepare the Salmon: Line a baking sheet with parchment paper for easy cleanup. Place the salmon filets on the baking sheet and drizzle each with olive oil. Rub the minced garlic over the filets and then season with dried dill, salt (if using), and freshly ground black pepper.
3. Add Lemon Slices: Arrange thin lemon slices over the top of each salmon filet. The lemon will not only add a bright flavor but also keep the fish moist while baking.
4. Bake the Salmon: Place the baking sheet in the preheated oven and bake the salmon for 12-15 minutes

or until the fish flakes easily with a fork. The exact cooking time may vary depending on the thickness of the filets.
5. Garnish and Serve: Once the salmon is cooked, remove it from the oven and transfer the filets to serving plates. Garnish with fresh parsley and additional lemon slices on the side.

Grilled Chicken Breast

Ingredients:

- 4 boneless, skinless chicken breasts (about 6 ounces each)
- 2 tablespoons olive oil
- Juice of 1 lemon
- 2 garlic cloves, minced
- 1 teaspoon dried rosemary (or fresh, if available)
- Salt (optional) and freshly ground black pepper to taste
- Fresh herbs like parsley or thyme for garnish (optional)

Instructions:

1. Prepare the Chicken: Begin by gently pounding the chicken breasts to an even thickness. This helps in cooking the chicken evenly throughout. Combine olive oil, lemon juice, minced garlic, dried rosemary, a dash of salt (optional), and black pepper in a small bowl.
2. Marinate: Place the chicken breasts in a shallow dish or a resealable plastic bag. Pour the marinade over the chicken, making sure each piece is well coated. Cover or seal and refrigerate for at least 30 minutes, or up to 4 hours for more flavor.
3. Preheat the Grill: Preheat your grill to medium-high heat. Ensure the grates are clean and lightly brush them with oil to prevent sticking.

4. Grill the Chicken: Remove the chicken from the marinade, letting any excess drip off. Place the chicken on the grill and cook for 6-7 minutes per side, or until the chicken is cooked through and reaches an internal temperature of 165°F (74°C). The cooking time may vary based on the thickness of the chicken breasts.
5. Rest and Serve: Once cooked, transfer the chicken breasts to a plate and cover loosely with foil. Let them rest for 5 minutes before serving. This allows the juices to redistribute, keeping the chicken moist and tender.
6. Garnish and Enjoy: Serve the grilled chicken breasts whole or sliced, garnished with fresh herbs if desired.

Conclusion

Congratulations on completing your journey through our Circadian diet guide! By investing the time to walk through these pages, you've taken a significant leap toward aligning your dietary habits with the natural rhythms of your body. This step is not just about adopting a new eating pattern; it's about enhancing your overall well-being and taking control of your health. We sincerely thank you for allowing us to be a part of this important transition in your life.

Understanding and implementing the principles of the Circadian diet marks the beginning of a profound transformation. This diet, grounded in the science of our internal biological clocks, is designed to optimize your body's natural processes. Eating in sync with your circadian rhythms can lead to remarkable benefits, including improved metabolic health, better sleep quality, and a decreased risk of various chronic diseases. It's a holistic approach that doesn't just change how you eat but potentially transforms how you feel, sleep, and live.

Implementing the Circadian diet is a commitment—a commitment to listen more attentively to your body and respond to its cues. It's normal to face challenges as you adjust your eating schedule and habits. These hurdles are part of the process, and overcoming them is what leads to growth and adaptation. Remember, it's not about perfection but progress. Each step you take towards aligning your eating habits with your circadian rhythm is a step toward better health.

We encourage you to approach this transition with patience and kindness towards yourself. Celebrate your successes, no matter how small they appear. Every meal that falls in harmony with your circadian rhythm is a milestone worth recognizing. And when things don't go as planned, extend yourself grace and compassion. Each new day brings another opportunity to reinforce your commitment to your health and well-being.

The beauty of the Circadian diet lies in its flexibility. It isn't a one-size-fits-all regimen but a framework that can be tailored to fit your unique lifestyle, preferences, and nutritional needs. This adaptability is what makes the Circadian diet a sustainable choice, capable of supporting your health goals in the long run.

As you move forward, stay curious and open to learning more about the fascinating interplay between nutrition and circadian biology. The field is continuously evolving, offering fresh insights into how we can further enhance our health through informed dietary choices. Keep experimenting, and don't hesitate to refine your approach as you gain new knowledge and experience.

You're not alone on this path. A vibrant community of individuals is exploring the Circadian diet, each with its own set of experiences and discoveries to share. Engaging with this community can offer invaluable support, motivation, and inspiration as you continue on your health and wellness journey.

Once again, we thank you for taking the time to explore the wonders of the Circadian diet. Your dedication to aligning your dietary habits with your body's natural rhythms is commendable. Here's to your health, happiness, and a harmonious relationship with your body's innate timing. Wishing you all the best as you continue to explore, learn, and grow on this rewarding path.

FAQ

What is the Circadian Diet?

The Circadian Diet is a nutritional approach that aligns your eating patterns with your body's circadian rhythms, or natural 24-hour cycle. It emphasizes consuming foods at times when your body is most biologically equipped to digest and metabolize them efficiently.

How does the Circadian Diet benefit health?

Following the Circadian Diet can lead to several health benefits, including improved metabolism, enhanced sleep quality, increased energy levels during the day, and potentially reduced risk of obesity and related chronic conditions. It works by syncing meal times with your body's internal clock, promoting optimal function.

Can I lose weight by following the Circadian Diet?

While the primary focus of the Circadian Diet is to promote overall health and well-being by aligning eating habits with circadian rhythms, many people find that it naturally leads to weight loss. This is often due to reduced late-night snacking and the more efficient metabolism of foods.

What does a typical day look like on the Circadian Diet?

A typical day on the Circadian Diet might involve eating a nutritious breakfast soon after waking up, enjoying a substantial lunch, and having a lighter dinner well before bedtime. Ideally, you should aim to eat your last meal at least 2-3 hours before going to sleep to align with circadian rhythms.

Are there any foods that are particularly encouraged or discouraged in the Circadian Diet?

The Circadian Diet doesn't strictly ban any specific foods but encourages whole, nutrient-dense foods that support your body's daily rhythms. Foods rich in fiber, protein, healthy fats, and antioxidants are recommended. Highly processed foods, sugary drinks, and excessive caffeine, especially later in the day, are discouraged.

How do I start following the Circadian Diet?

To start following the Circadian Diet, begin by adjusting your meal times to better align with daylight hours—eating larger meals earlier in the day and reducing food intake as evening approaches. Gradually shift your dinner time earlier and aim for a fasting window of 12-14 hours overnight.

What should I do if my schedule doesn't allow for an early dinner?

If your schedule makes it challenging to have an early dinner, try to make your evening meal as light as possible and focus on easily digestible foods. Also, maintain consistency in your meal timing from day to day, as regularity can help support your circadian rhythms even if perfect timing isn't always possible.

References and Helpful Links

Munshi, P. (2023, April 16). Circadian diet: Eat THESE food items to keep your health right. English Jagran.
https://english.jagran.com/lifestyle/circadian-diet-eat-these-foods-items-to-keep-your-heath-right-10073677

Intermittent fasting and circadian rhythm: 10 tips to make intermittent fasting work for you. (n.d.). NDTV.com.
https://www.ndtv.com/health/intermittent-fasting-and-circadian-rhythm-10-tips-to-bring-fasting-in-line-with-your-bodys-biologica-2135654

Branch, K. (2019, January 16). The best weight loss diet comes down to When—Not just What—You eat. Vogue.
https://www.vogue.com/article/best-diet-to-lose-weight-intermittent-fasting-circadian-rhythms-gut-health-skin

Vyasan, N., & Vyasan, N. (2023, April 15). Circadian Diet: 5 Foods to Eat and Avoid to optimise your health. News18.
https://www.news18.com/lifestyle/circadian-diet-5-foods-to-eat-and-avoid-to-optimise-your-health-7550881.html

What is the circadian rhythm diet? How to eat with the sun. (2019, February 21). TODAY.com.
https://www.today.com/health/what-circadian-rhythm-diet-how-eat-sun-t149238

Thrive Natural Medicine Soquel. (2021, July 15). The Circadian Rhythm Diet - Thrive Natural medicine. Thrive Natural Medicine. https://thrivenatmed.com/naturopathic-medicine-soquel/circadian-rhythm-diet/

How to Eat in Harmony with Your Circadian Rhythms. (n.d.). Kripalu. https://kripalu.org/resources/how-eat-harmony-your-circadian-rhythms

Smith, M., MA. (2024, February 28). How to fall asleep fast and sleep Better. HelpGuide.org. https://www.helpguide.org/articles/sleep/getting-better-sleep.htm

Circadian diet another form of intermittent fasting. (2021, October 1). UCLA Health. https://www.uclahealth.org/news/circadian-diet-another-form-of-intermittent-fasting#:~:text=In%20the%20circadian%20diet%2C%20you,midnight%20raids%20on%20the%20fridge.

www.ingramcontent.com/pod-product-compliance
Lightning Source LLC
LaVergne TN
LVHW021230080526
838199LV00089B/5985